Weight

Loss

Hope

By Arnoux Goran

1st Edition

totalhealthmastery

For general information on our other products and services or to submit a book for publishing please visit us at our website www.THMastery.com

ISBN: 9 780979 679308

This book is dedicated to all of those who have tried to lose weight and failed, and to those who never even thought they stood a chance. You CAN be thin!

Table of Contents

Foreword

By Ms. America Fitness '06 -'07

Kardena Pauza

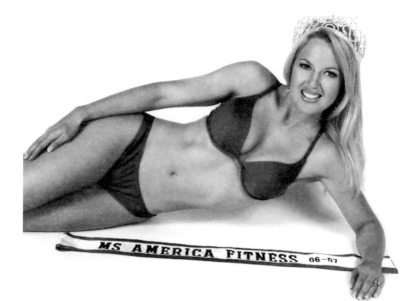

Weight Loss Hope

This is a life changing book period! It's an easy to follow step by step process to effortlessly make incredible changes in your life. We were meant to have abundant energy, have a lean beautiful body, radiant skin and think positive thoughts. We were meant to live without disease and without sickness. Because of Arnoux's challenging & courageous life journey he has been inspired to share his knowledge of how to be healthy with the world and to teach others how to lose weight and feel amazing! Many medical experts don't believe nutrition is the key to health and longevity. Arnoux will share through experience and seeing results how proper nutrition can regenerate the body to perfect health. Many people fight and struggle with their weight, they drag themselves through their day with no energy. This suffering can be overcome by following the powerful principles Arnoux has outlined in this life changing book! We all know there is a better way to live!

We realize that there is a strong body-emotion-mind connection and the way to bring about a healthy body is to also address the emotional & mental aspect of ourselves. As we start to make dietary and lifestyle changes we come up against situations or feelings that may stop us from reaching our health goals. I find that Arnoux's powerful process for clearing blocks is amazing and effective. By using his quick and easy method of clearing unwanted thoughts and emotions you can begin to empower and inspire yourself to stay on the path you were initially excited about - losing weight and being super healthy.

Many of us are very busy and time is a factor when we think about what we are going to eat. I've found that lack of preparation is one of the biggest reasons my clients gain weight, don't get results & drop off their program. Arnoux gives time saving healthy tips and recipes that will make preparing food quick and easy. When you are on the go these delicious meals can go with you!

I am a certified personal trainer and the owner of Edge Personal Training. I personally use the methods Arnoux shares and I teach them to my clients. My clients are so happy because the processes assist them in reaching their weight goals and they are mentally & emotionally much happier.

Thank you Arnoux for the wonderful work you do!
Kardena Pauza

Contact Kardena at www.edgetrainers.com

Preface – A Reason to be Inspired

Dear Oprah,

How I got from picture before (warning –terrible photo's on display – I'm sure they were taken by some rag tabloid) what I call my 'sumo wrestler' picture, to after, what I call my yahoo!! — look at me now picture, is an amazing, amazing journey, and one that I would like to share with all of you.

My name is Samara Christy; I am age 57 and I have been, like many others, overweight for most of my life. As I got older, my inability to lose weight got increasingly worse. I would try diet after diet with my friends, and they would lose 30-40 pounds and I would lose about ten. Then in a few months, I would return to my original weight and then over a period of about six months I would gain an additional ten to twenty pounds. What made matters worse, was I had been a health care practitioner for more than 25 years and I was truly embarrassed and humiliated by my inability to lose weight. My heart would break when my clients, all meaning to be helpful, would hand me yet another diet to try. In retaliation, I threatened to wear to the Healing

Center, my super size tee shirt over my 200lb plus body that said, 'I fought anorexia and won.' I often made jokes about my weight in an attempt to cover up my pain. When my husband Ken, fiancé then, and I were first dating, he took me on a wonderful vacation to Puerto Vallarta. We had a beautiful time as we sat on the beach and sipped margaritas while we watched the sun set so magnificently as only Puerto Vallarta is famous for. I was in love, and as my fiancé and I looked dreamily into each other's eyes while we ate our sumptuous dinner, I shared my concerns that what we were eating was more than I usually ate and that I would probably gain weight on this trip. Ken looked at me incredulously, and blurted out, "that's impossible." You see, to support me in losing weight, we would order one lunch or one dinner and ask for another plate so that we could split our meal. In fact, we would split all our meals on that trip.

Because I did not speak the language and Ken spoke enough Spanish, we agreed that he would carry all the cash and pay for everything. So my fiancé knew everything that I ate because he was the only one with the money to buy anything. When we returned from our vacation, we both weighed in on our first morning home. He had lost eight pounds and my worst fears had been realized, I had gained five. My fiancé apologized to me saying that he had a confession to make. That all those nights that we were dating and that we had been splitting our meals, he had just assumed that I must be eating when I went home from our dates. Ouch! That really hurt! Don't get me wrong, my fiancé truly loved me in spite of my weight, but as you know, unless you have lived it, you don't fully understand it.

Finally, I just gave up (picture A) and resigned myself that this was going to be my fate. I still continued to pray, "God you have had an answer for everything else in my life, why not the weight? There just has got to be an answer -- somewhere?" Soon a group of clients started coming to me, many of them like me, over 50 and overweight. This group was in a ten-week program and they all lost about 25 – 30 lbs or more in three months. Well that really got my attention and I wanted to meet this guy who taught that class. His name is Arnoux (pronounced 'are know') Goran. He was 27 years old at the time and looked about 19. I began having second thoughts. What could this kid teach me? Then I remembered my wonderfully thin clients. I immediately arranged to meet with him. Arnoux shared with me his amazing story of how he had come to create this program. It was hard to imagine that this handsome, articulate man was born to deaf parents who suffered from drug addiction. As a result of an incredibly tumultuous childhood, Arnoux's health was seriously compromised. Though he was never overweight, he shared with me that his doctors didn't give him long to live. As Arnoux went from doctor to doctor desperately looking for help, he finally discovered the secrets of health he shares in his Total Health Mastery programs and went on to heal every single one of his many aliments. Then he went on to teach what he knew to help others by creating the Total Health Mastery seminars, and making himself available as a Professional Health Consultant. His clients began to get radiantly healthy, and his hopelessly overweight and over 50 women began to lose weight and to keep it off.

I decided to give his program a try, after all what did I have to lose (about 80 pounds to be exact) so I plunged headlong into the information, and to my shock, I too lost 10 pounds the very first month. What happened next was even more amazing. My energy just shot through the roof. My food before, though healthy food, left me feeling tired all the time. I know the experts preach exercise is key, but how do you exercise when you only have enough energy to barely get though your day? After a month on the program, I had energy to burn and I began going to Curves where at first I could only get half way around their circuit. Six months into it, the Curves owner offered me a job, telling me people asked when I worked out because they found me supportive and inspiring and they wanted to work out with me.

To my delight, the Total Health Mastery program worked. I lost 50 lbs in the first five and ½ months and I am still losing. I am 5'4" and I weighed 213 lbs, and I weighed 163 lbs when the after picture was taken. Not only did I lose the weight but I am in glowing health. To my amazement the loose skin that many women who have lost a lot of weight have to have surgically removed, didn't happen to me or any of the other course participants that I met. We are all living proof that these principles of health work.

However, about two months into my health program, the emotional issues that were keeping me from losing weight did come up, big time! I owe many thanks to Arnoux, my Professional Health Consultant, who helped me and encouraged me through that terrible, terrible time. You see, I didn't lose weight like normal people while doing this program. Most people would lose about 2 to 2 ½ pounds a week. I would go for about three weeks without losing any weight. Then I would feel a tremor in my body that would last for about two days followed by my getting emotionally hysterical. It seemed my body was fighting for its life not to lose the pounds. Then the very next day, I would lose about six pounds all at once. You see, I had been sexually assaulted at a very young age. I was kidnapped and assaulted near my school at age 15 by a man who posed as a cop. I have done a lot of talk therapy over the years to help heal this trauma, but I soon discovered that the shock from this episode was somehow locked in my body. Arnoux developed a process called The 7-Steps to Reprogramming Yourself, it together with the help of EMDR, rapid eye movement therapy released me from the terrible fear that was coming up as my weight, my protection, began to drop.

Arnoux's process is designed to handle the emotional reasons people can't lose weight.

I am forever grateful to Total Health Mastery for introducing me to the information that not only helped me to lose my weight for the very last time, but for offering me a way of life that put me on a journey that would ultimately lead to my letting go of the baggage I had been carrying for more than 42 years.

Oprah, many of your famous guests, Demi Moore for one, as well as many other well known celebrities, like Alicia Silverstone, Woody Harrelson, Carol Alt, and Donna Karan are serious health advocates. Not only do they know that this program can manage their weight but it can seriously restore their health. Please investigate Arnoux's programs, starting with his book on weight loss Weight Loss Hope, I guarantee you will be amazed.

Well that's my story Oprah. Thank you so much for listening.

Sincerely, Samara Christy, Health Care Practitioner
Scottsdale, Arizona

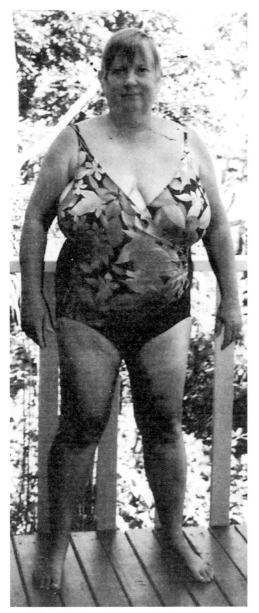

Samara Before

Samara After

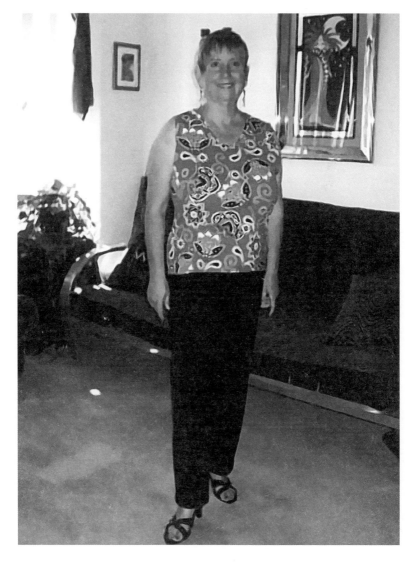

Chapter One
Why You Can Succeed Now

In this book you will discover why you can succeed now even if you never have before and little known secrets of nutrition that can help you **lose a pound a day** and reach your ideal weight mixed with the best recipes for weight loss, health, energy and beauty. Learn the world's most advanced scientific information explained in simple, understandable terms how **you** can lose weight and have your ideal body.

Finally, understand WHY you don't lose weight and how you can. This breakthrough book will inform you of the simple yet extremely effective secrets of nutrition and how your body works.

You will learn multiple weight loss facts that will allow you to lose as much as one pound per day safely and effectively. **These facts are scientific** and you will learn the sources AND how to use the information for you. You'll also receive several delicious weight loss recipes including *Arnoux's famous Chocolate shake, which actually causes weight loss!*

Check out this testimonial:

"I told Arnoux that I wanted to lose about 10 lbs but that I didn't want to make any major changes in my lifestyle or start exercising. Did he have a secret for me? Surprisingly, he said he did. He taught me about how metabolism is created in the body nutritionally and how the two ESSENTIAL nutrients for creating metabolism and weight loss are not part of the standard American diet. He also taught me that the number seven prescribed drug in America is a drug that affects metabolism. I tried his suggestion for getting one of the nutrients in my body, the more important one, and I was really surprised at what happened. I called Arnoux 10 days after we spoke to tell him the good news, I had lost 10lbs!"   - Sean Hutchinson, San Diego, CA

People often spend hundreds or thousands of dollars on weight loss drugs, pills, programs and more that don't work. Find out what's really causing your weight loss challenges and address them finally with this book, *Weight Loss Hope.*

A client of mine once gave me 300 books on weight loss in exchange for a one-hour consultation. I got a bad deal. Not a single book contained any information worth putting into action, which is why after spending over $6,000 on those books and hundreds of hours reading them she still had no idea how to lose weight. I was able to tell her how in less than 60 minutes. Thankfully you won't have to read thousands of pages of books to learn how to lose weight and keep it off. The guidelines are in this book.

My name is Arnoux (are-know) Goran and **I was once diagnosed with several "incurable" diseases and told that I would certainly die.** These diseases included: arthritis, fibromyalgia, chronic fatigue syndrome, anemia, hypoglycemia, adrenal failure, ulcers, hemorrhoids, candida, asthma, severe allergies, sinusitis, rhinitis and more. I was always getting the flu, bronchitis or worse. I was often in the emergency room with a bad infection. I didn't breathe through my nose for over five years. I was in constant pain, totally exhausted and couldn't remember things I read so I finally had to quit the pre-med program that I was in and pray for answers. I had already quit working and teaching martial arts. Although my body was done, my sprit wasn't willing to give up.

I didn't believe any of my doctors when they said, "you're already on the strongest medication," or "there's nothing we can do for you," or "you're just going to have to learn to live with the pain." I just thought that they didn't know how I could heal myself. After trying all types of allopathic doctors (western medical doctors), Chinese doctors, naturopathic doctors, chiropractors, massage therapists, acupuncturists, energy healers and more I finally just started praying.

It wasn't long before I discovered that **the source of** *physical* **health is the diet.** We've all heard the saying, "you are what you eat" but I never took it literally. I was in phenomenal shape outwardly as a black belt and instructor under one of the greatest martial arts masters in the world, except that inwardly I was dying. All of the best exercise in the world didn't make me healthy. What made me healthy was a shift in my diet.

After changing my diet it took *only six months* for me to discover perfect health.

YES, perfect health!

I had nothing wrong with me. No pain in my body. No blood in the toilet. No exhaustion. No bleeding gums. No runny noses. No swollen joints. No dandruff, No dry skin, No body odor or even bad breath! I was totally healed just by eating the foods that the human body is designed to eat.

Unfortunately, everything I was eating, which I'll share with you later, went totally against what I already knew, or thought I knew about health and nutrition. So I began studying by reading everything I could. I discovered one fact that changed my life; and it may change yours too.

Here it is:

The nutritional education in America in public schools and even for physical therapists is provided by the National Dairy Council with the support of the meat and egg industries.

Please don't take my word for it. Go to your local school right now and look at their nutritional materials. They say "National Dairy Council" on them.

The National Dairy Council has been the source of health education in America since 1915. As of today that's almost 100 years! There probably isn't an American alive who went to school before then.

This means that everything you learned in school, as well as learned from your family, friends, peers, teachers and even the media was National Dairy Council information.

This was shocking to me and even more surprising was when I started reading medical journals, scientific journals and books written by brilliant doctors I discovered what the studies actually say; I found out that almost everything we have been taught doesn't work in the real world at all.

At first I felt very angry to read that fact in *Diet for a New America* by John Robbins. After the anger subsided I was actually very grateful that I became enlightened by this very simple yet important truth. Everything I thought I knew and most everything that pretty much everyone else I know thinks they know about health is totally inaccurate. Thankfully, my mind was now opened up to discovering completely anew what really works in regards to health and of course, weight loss.

John Robbins, the author of *Diet for a New America,* has an interesting story. Heir to the Baskin and Robbins ice cream empire, he saw his uncle Mr. Baskins die of a heart attack and suspected that ice cream was the cause. After reading many, many studies he published a book about his findings on the truth about nutrition, and gave up his empire. Although his book only covers some of what we need to know about health and nutrition, it opened up my eyes and my mind to new ideas.

As I continued to read book after book by great doctors who have no problem helping people heal themselves of various illnesses I began to see patterns. There are principles of health and healing that are true for everyone and when applied consistently will allow ANYONE to be healthy, lose weight or create the body of their dreams.

I've dedicated my entire life to developing a complete training program for health education so that no one has to suffer the way that I did ever again. Over the last nine years I have enjoyed perfect health and my research and experience have taught me a great deal. I have developed the educational program that I dreamed of *The Solution Weekend Seminar, The Total Health Mastery 10-Week Seminar* and *The Total Health Mastery Series* which includes the information on weight loss in this book and so much more.

As my mission to create a world of health for everyone unfolded I realized that I needed to study emotional and mental healing as well. Emotions are chemicals that live in your cells and they begin to come to the surface when you start to release the poisons accumulated in your body, which naturally happens when you change your diet to a healthier one.

As the oldest child of two deaf parents who suffered with a horrible cocaine addiction for over 12 years I had quite a bit of emotional trauma. Thank God my parents are both clean and sober and have been for over 10 years and are accomplishing great things in life. But for me, there remained a journey of emotional healing that became a driving factor in me studying the mind and emotions, beyond what I learned as a black belt and martial arts instructor or athlete growing up.

Years of research, prayers and trial and error finally resulted in the creation of a new method of releasing old emotions and reprogramming the subconscious mind, or the belief system, *permanently*. A technique that is undoubtedly one of the fastest and easiest methods that exists in the world today. And the basics of how to do it are in this book! The technique is called *The 7-Steps to Reprogramming Yourself*, and it will change your life forever to master and use this simple yet powerful technique.

I then was led to truly understand the nature of addiction. Beyond my parent's own drug problems, I had an addiction that I couldn't shake as well. Food Addiction. Even after learning to release old emotions as they came up, and having without any doubt a clear understanding of how the body works, what foods truly create optimal health in the body and so on, I still had a food addiction. So I dedicated myself to resolving that problem, and created *How to Overcome Addictions Without Willpower*. Ultimately, it's a program on how to have zero cravings. No cravings means no addiction in simplest terms. Some of the basics are in this book as well.

I also faced another challenge, cleansing reactions. When people heal their bodies, which includes losing weight, toxins come out of the body and if not done properly this cleansing process can be very uncomfortable. Every book I read and every teacher I studied under taught me that cleansing reactions such as fevers, headaches, chills, fatigue, nausea, skin breakouts, diarrhea and even vomiting are all part of cleansing and detoxifying the body. I decided there must be an easier way and through great study with a focus on finding the easier way created *How to Cleanse the Body Without Cleansing Reactions*, which can be found in our trainings available via recording, teleconference or in person.

Naturally, it's in my book *How to Cleanse Your Body: Without Cleansing Reactions*! Yes, there really is tar and other scary things in you and you'll be shocked *and* thrilled when it comes out.

The combination of study and application for many years with a total focus in my life on creating the most advanced, most useful educational training on health has created a program that has mind blowing results. You've read a few of the testimonials already in this book, and believe me, that's only a fraction of them.

Many people in this country and around the world are facing weight loss issues. Over 65% of Americans are overweight and over 30% are obese. Childhood diabetes is growing at an alarming rate with no end in sight. The disease of obesity is rampant and yes it's disease. It's not easy to be overweight, and the pain people feel from being overweight calls to me and that's why this book has been written. To help you, whoever you are, to lose weight, even if you've tried everything and nothing has worked, finally, you will understand how to lose weight and keep it off. You can lose weight too!

Before we get into the knowledge, I would like to share with you a few more stories from people that I've shared this information with who took it and ran with it.

"Five months after meeting Arnoux while he was teaching How to Overcome Addictions Without Willpower" I have lost forty pounds, reversed fibromyalgia, depression and chronic fatigue syndrome, gotten off of all pain, depression and sleep medications that I was on for 17 years, begun outrigger canoeing, cleaned and organized my whole house! I am a full time nurse and have been in the medical field for over twenty years. During all of this time I never learned as much as I did in *The Total Health Mastery 10-Week Seminar.* I tried program after program to heal myself all the while my doctors were telling me that all that could be done for the pain and exhaustion was to give me more drugs. They said I was depressed and gave me more drugs. All of the other "alternative" programs I tried didn't work. I tried many for months at a time before I finally gave up. Arnoux's program worked for me right away. I saw results and that inspired me to keep going. I am so grateful for Arnoux!!!"

- Stephanie Grainger, Nurse, Orange County, CA

"I was on a weight loss program that was working well for me. I had lost fifty pounds on my own but had hit a wall. Arnoux put me on a program and in thirty days I lost thirty-five pounds. My doctor was so happy. He put me on an EKG machine and it turns out my heart and blood pressure medication was no longer necessary! I highly recommend Arnoux's programs and the principles he teaches. It works."

- George R. Adams, Attorney, Washington DC

"I have lost over 44 pounds, got rid of my carpal tunnel pain and need a lot less sleep than ever before. I also shared this information with my mother and she too lost over 30 pounds, got rid of the swelling in her legs and completely eliminated her need for insulin! She was taking four shots of insulin a day and was told by her doctor that she no longer needs them. It's a true blessing to have my mother and I be healthier then we could have ever imagined in a matter of months and it was easy. I am grateful to Arnoux and Total Health Mastery for making such a difference for us."

– Carmen Sanchez, Chicago, IL

Should I go on with the testimonials? There are many more. Lots and lots of people are losing 30 pounds in 30 days on a program I gave them or that they created themselves after taking *The Total Health Mastery 10-Week Seminar*. My own brother lost 55 pounds in 10 months on a very simple program - this was AFTER he got his black belt. I think I've teased you enough, let me show you how to create yourself as one of these testimonials. Even if all you want to lose is five pounds or 25 pounds before a wedding. This book will show you the path towards achieving your personal weight loss goals.

Chapter Two
You Are More Than Just A Body

To achieve your goals in any area of life, including weight loss or healing an illness, we must address all four parts of you: Physical, emotional, mental and spiritual. Most people only address one area and then wonder why they aren't getting results. If you can address your whole self: physical, emotional, mental and spiritual, then you can have the success you desire. I will show you how to do that.

Let me break it all down for you on two simple pages - and then fill in the details.

Physical

To have perfect health on the physical level you only need two things: Put in all of the essential nutrients and remove all of the toxins.

Emotional

Emotions are chemicals and live in the cells of your body. Emotions of anger, sadness and fear are very toxic to the body and need to be released. Stuffing your emotions does not make you tough, only foolish. A true warrior has the courage to feel and release their feelings using advanced technology that I will share with you later in this book.

Mental

You have beliefs that don't support you that must be changed. Most of these beliefs are subconscious, so you need to re-program yourself. This includes changing your self-image or the picture in your mind of what you look like. You also need an environment that supports you.

Spiritual (or Energetic)

The human body is made of spirit or energy as well. Whatever religious or spiritual traditions you are a part of, use them to help create your weight loss and health success.

Chapter Three
The Physical Body and Secret #1

To have perfect health on the physical level only requires two things. Put in all of the essential nutrients and remove all of the toxins. That's it!

There is a famous experiment called the *Chicken Heart Experiment* that illustrates this principle found in a great book called *Cleanse and Purify Thyself book* 1 by Dr. Richard Anderson and in Anthony Robbins' audio program (the best selling audio program of all time) *Personal Power.*

Researchers were able to keep a chicken's heart alive for 29 years simply by providing the proper nutrients and removing the toxins it naturally produced. When they forgot to change the water for a few days, it died. Chickens only live to be 11.

Your body is the same way. We need to put the nutrients in and get the toxins out for it to work right. Being overweight isn't a sign of being lazy or gluttonous as much as it is a sign of having a body that is out of balance. You haven't done anything wrong; you just didn't know up until now how to properly take care of your body. Once you do, everything will change for you. Your self-esteem will go up, you'll feel empowered, people will notice you and you'll be very happy about it.

Before I give you the basics of proper eating, let me give you the two secrets of weight loss on the physical level that will work to help you lose weight regardless of what your diet is or how much you exercise.

Secret #1

Metabolism – The Rate at Which Your Body Burns Calories

When it comes to weight loss there are many important nutrients, and there are two major nutrients that are especially important because they affect your body's **metabolism.**

The gland in your body that controls metabolism, the rate at which your body burns calories, is called the thyroid. No matter how much you exercise if your thyroid doesn't work properly, you'll have little or no metabolism, and not lose weight. Thyroid medication is the number seven prescribed drug in America - that's because the two nutrients the thyroid needs to make the hormones that cause metabolism in your body are non-existent in the Standard American Diet or SAD.

Those two nutrients are saturated fat and iodine.

Wait a minute. Are you, Arnoux, saying there is no saturated fat in the American diet, one high in beef, which is 72% saturated fat?

Yes and no.

Any saturated fat that is processed, cooked or oxidized is not usable by the human body. Your liver cannot digest it, so your thyroid can't use it for the most part. All it does is clog up your blood stream, make you acidic and eventually can kill you. Your body can only effectively use fats that are digestible, which means fresh, living or raw, in their natural state. A wonderful man named Udo Erasmus spent six years of his life studying and reading every single scientific study EVER done on fats. After all of this study he wrote a book on his findings, a book about everything we as a civilization know about fats, *The Fats that Heal, the Fats that Kill.* And it really came down to one basic thing - if they are processed (heated or oxidized) they cannot be used and are actually very toxic to the body. Fats are very, very important for health and most people are deficient. Dr. David Jubb, PhD reports in his book, *LifeFood Recipe Book* that 100% of Americans tested are deficient in essential fats.

Do you live in America? If so, there is a pretty good chance, about 100%, that you are deficient in essential fats, which are Omega 3 and Omega 6. I go into much more detail about fats, why they are so crucial to health and how so **many health challenges are caused by fat deficiency** including brain chemistry issues in our trainings and my book *The 11 Must Haves: The Essential Nutrients Your Body Needs.* Find them at www.THMastery.com. For now just know that you need raw or living saturated fat to fuel your thyroid and create metabolism. This is a HUGE, HUGE, HUGE secret!

If you just put good saturated fats, or *any good* fats into your body you will begin to get your thyroid on track and producing more metabolism. You can lose weight by eating food that is delicious! You always knew it was true, and now you have found out how!

Please note this will work ONLY if your metabolism is slow. It's incredibly common in America, but not everyone has a slow metabolism.

Sources of Good Saturated Fat

- Young Coconuts - Not the brown ones but rather the white ones wrapped in plastic found at the Asian markets or health food stores. Learn to open them by watching *The SuperStyle Diet Recipe Class Video* or by searching YouTube.com for "how to open a young coconut".

- Avocados - There are 76 different types of avocados worldwide.

- Olives - Stored in glass jars, alive or raw, not in aluminum cans as they are cooked.

- Nuts - Fresh, living or raw only. If it's roasted it's not alive or useable anymore! Please note that all Almonds in America are now pasteurized, ask your grocer for details.

- Seeds - Living only. Again, if it's roasted it's not alive anymore.

- Oils - Organic, cold pressed, in a dark bottle, and extra virgin for olive oil. Bariani's is by far the best olive oil, found on our website. Be sure to try flax, hemp or Udo's oil for maximum results.

All foods including your good fats must be organic if possible. Organic means natural. If it is not organic it is called commercial which means it's grown with seeds that may be genetically modified **which may modify YOUR DNA**.

Commercial foods are also grown in soil with toxic waste used for fertilizer and are heavily sprayed with chemicals that are variations of Vietnam war chemical warfare, are totally devoid of nutrients and basically not good for your body. If you're wondering why **America is LAST in the world in health but spends more money on healthcare than anyone else** - you have a couple of hints: false information and poor food quality.

When you look at other countries, they eat meat, pastries and other "junk" foods, but they aren't nearly as sick or overweight as we are. In *Cleanse and Purify Thyself* by Dr. Richard Anderson you'll find evidence stating that America ranks last, DEAD LAST of the 100 industrialized nations that participate in the regular global study of health. We are the most unhealthy and overweight country by far, and it's unfortunate because we are also the richest. The cause of this problem lies heavily in our poor food quality. For example, our meat is banned from Europe. Our meat is *illegal* in Europe as part of 53 other companies! See *Mad Cowboy* by Howard Lyman for details (MadCowboy.com). Please eat organic food as much as possible if you truly want to be healthy and thin. Organic is a code word for hot and sexy, if it's not organic it means fat, overweight, obese, sick and tired.

You may be wondering how much good fat to eat? AS MUCH AS YOU WANT! Fat is not bad for you. Living fats do not contain cholesterol. Cholesterol is made in the liver of animals. As far as I know, I've never heard of an avocado with a liver. Have you? Living fats will make you lose weight. Remember, fat is higher in calories than proteins and carbohydrates so watch your body, you may go overboard with excitement! If you gain weight (very rare, maybe 1 in 100) you may want to focus more on oils rather than other fat sources.

Every single testimonial that you have read in this book included eating healthy living, raw, natural fats. They are essential for health AND weight loss. Everything you have learned about fat is wrong. Sorry, but it is! Fat is not the devil. Fat is not bad for you. Bad fats are bad for you and good fats are good for you. YOU NEED GOOD FATS TO LOSE WEIGHT. Generally, the only time you can eat too many good fats is if you're emotionally eating and using them to stuff emotions. We'll address emotional eating in Chapter Seven.

Try it out! Just try three tablespoons of flax oil every morning, that can't possibly hurt.

You may lose 1 lb a day as so many others have! Go for it! What have you got to lose?

Well…maybe a few pounds! You're now on your way to your ideal body. Remember, keep an open mind. These concepts have worked for so many of my seminar participants and they can work for you as well.

The Other Nutrient For The Thyroid

Iodine. It's iodine that also fuels the thyroid, which is found most abundantly in sea vegetables, especially kelp. You can find kelp tablets at your local health food store. Kelp is good for you in many ways, so it won't hurt to take it. Enjoy.

Chapter Three Inspired Actions

Choose any one or more of the following *Inspired Actions:*

- Purchase a bottle of flax oil from your local health food store and take at least three tablespoons per day for one month.

- Purchase a Young Coconut and learn how to open it. Enjoy the amazing water and meat.

- Replace one bad fat meal, generally one high in animal products with a good fat meal, at least once per week. (For recipes see www.THMastery.com "Free Tools".)

- Read *Coconut Cures or The Healing Miracles of Coconut Oil* by Dr. Bruce Fife, ND and learn that young coconuts pull the plaque off your arteries!

- Redeem your FREE copy of *The Awakening* audio training ($97 value), see page 90 for details.

Chapter Four
The Physical Body and Secret #2

Now that you know how to create metabolism let's go on to the other secret of weight loss on the physical level: removing toxins.

Secret #2

The Human Body Stores Toxins in the Fat Cells

Here is one of the biggest, most unknown yet important secrets of weight loss: your body stores toxins in your fat cells and generally WILL NOT BREAK DOWN THE FAT CELLS UNLESS IT CAN REMOVE THE TOXINS, which in most cases it can't. You can exercise all day every day and live on 1,000 calories a day and you won't lose those last 20 pounds or that cellulite unless the toxins can come out of your body. All mammals store toxins in their fat cells. That's why beef has 14 times more pesticides in it than commercially grown food, because the cows keep eating soy and corn and other foods that are highly sprayed and keep storing those toxins in their fat cells. Even lean meats are high in fat, they are at least 50% fat most of the time. Look it up in *Diet for A New America* by John Robbins. If you do force your body to lose weight through exercise or surgeries, your skin may be left sagging as well as your elimination organs may become overloaded with toxins.

How do we eliminate toxins?

Simple. I will give you the two basic principles for eliminating toxins, the foundation for my book *How to Cleanse Your Body: Without Cleansing Reaction!,* a system which is revolutionary and totally original. Once you know these principles you will be able to do it - although the details that I cover in The Total Health Mastery Live Seminars are very important as well - many people lost weight just using these basics.

The two principles of removing toxins are: Create elimination through bowel movements and supply the body with minerals. That's it!

The Basics Of Creating Elimination

- Drink a lot of water. Not tap! Try a gallon of spring water every day for two weeks and see how you feel!
- Take probiotics
- Eat foods high in fiber, especially organic fresh fruits and vegetables. Incidentally organic is only more expensive when you compare apples to apples dipped in wax (yes commercial apples are dipped in wax to give them the glow). But when you compare doctor bills, health insurance costs, the cost of an illness, and the cost of feeling sick or being overweight, and most importantly the TASTE, organic is WAY cheaper. I didn't like many vegetables or even avocados until I tried organic foods. Commercial foods are generally tasteless in comparison.

- Drink a fiber shake.

- Take herbs to create elimination.

- Do enemas or colon hydro-therapy.

- Exercise (cardio) although exercise isn't nearly as important as nutrition for health and weight loss, it is important. It makes you breathe and breathing moves the lymphatic fluid in your body, which carries the wastes away from your cells and into the colon to be removed. That's why cardiovascular exercise is by far the best for weight loss. It also helps to take 10 deep breaths in and out through the nose to the low stomach three times per day.

- Do an intestinal cleanse.

How to properly create elimination is an entire class or book, but the basics above should help. The best way to eliminate quickly is to do an intestinal cleanse. People almost always lose one pound a day or more on a good intestinal cleanse if they have the weight to lose. People who are underweight gain weight because their assimilation improves. If you want to learn more about cleansing please register for our trainings by calling 1-877-680-8200 or visiting us at www.THMastery.com. You can attend live in person in Southern California or via teleconference, audio CD or on-line recording from anywhere in the world.

Most of the people who lost 30 pounds in 30 days did it while doing a fantastic intestinal cleanse. They improved their health so dramatically by getting such a large amount of toxins out very fast that they couldn't help but lose weight as a by product. Many people did the cleansing to get healthy, not lose weight and the weight loss was just an added benefit. I'll share some examples:

"I had acid reflux disease so badly that I couldn't sleep at night. I slept between three hours and thirty minutes each night. It was just a matter of the exhaustion overtaking the pain. My doctors already had me on the strongest medication and said there was nothing they could do. A friend recommended Arnoux. He put me on a 30 day cleanse with a HUGE amount of nutritional supplements. By the end of the 30 days I was sleeping eight hours per day, was off all medications and was completely out of pain. I also lost 35 pounds and started exercising because I finally felt like it."
- Rich Freedman, Business Consultant, Santa Fe, NM

"During *The Total Health Mastery 10-Week Seminar* I decided to do a cleanse. It was an eight-day cleanse and I lost 20 pounds and my skin looked amazing! I didn't have any cleansing reactions at all, which I found were common with my friends and co-workers who didn't have the benefit of Arnoux's information on how to cleanse without cleansing reactions."

- Jose Wantland, Massage Therapist, Orange County, CA

"I'm not the greatest student but I did do a cleanse during The Total Health Mastery Seminar and I was amazed that after four days the cellulite on my legs was totally gone! I had tried everything to get rid of it and that last five nasty pounds that just wouldn't go. With the cleanse, gone! Yes!"

- Allyson Meacham, Orange County, CA

Cleansing is something that everyone can benefit from. Anyone who says otherwise would probably also tell you that you can't lose weight, that you're already on the strongest medications and there's nothing that can be done for you. Please don't listen. Trust your heart. Trust your instincts. You *can* lose weight "and" keep it off! You *can* feel great.

Chapter Four Inspired Actions

Choose any one or more of the following *Inspired Actions:*

- Drink 1 gallon of spring water every day for 2 weeks

- Purchase a Health Cleanz kit, the best at home colon hydro-therapy kit. (www.THMastery.com)

- Read *How to Cleanse the Body: Without Cleansing Reactions!* (*www.THMastery.com*) and do an intestinal cleanse.

- Hire a Professional Health Consultant to help guide you and support you in achieving your weight loss goals (www.THMastery.com)

Chapter Five
Minerals

Your body needs minerals to remove toxins. It needs it for many more functions than you can imagine. Minerals are the number two component of your body, right after water. They are the key to good health physically along with the other 10 essential nutrients and are essential for weight loss. YOUR BODY CANNOT REMOVE TOXINS WITHOUT THE MINERALS TO PROCESS THEM.

If you want to lose weight you need to put A LOT of minerals into your body. The American diet is deficient of minerals, even if it's organic. Soil depletion has made the food mineral deficient. Commercial food has very little in it as far as minerals are concerned and this even includes vegetables.

The body uses alkaline (PH Balanced) minerals to neutralize the toxins, which are acidic (Not PH Balanced), so then they can be removed safely. No minerals = no toxin removal = no fat breakdown = no results!
Lots of minerals = lots of toxin removal = lots of fat breakdown = total joy!

Sources of Minerals

I have an entire course on minerals within *The Total Health Mastery 10-Week Seminar.* I also cover minerals in my book *The 11 Must Haves: The Essential Nutrients Your Body Needs.* I'm going to give you the basics here, which is plenty to get started and lose lots of weight fast.

- Organic vegetable juice (cucumber, celery and apple is a great base). The best juicers can be found at (www.THMastery.com.)

- Wild foods like algae's, sea vegetables, wild herbs and Amazon Rainforest Herbs found at (www.THMastery.com.)

- Mineral Broth: 3 stalks of celery, slice of apple, slice of lemon, 3 potatoes and one handful of greens all chopped in a big pot of water and simmer for 30 min - 2 hours, plus. Drink the broth. Recommended optional for flavor: Garlic, green onions, ginger, hot peppers, cilantro, oregano, basil, tomato, sea vegetables and other herbs or spices. It will last for four days refrigerated.

- Alfalfa Tablets

- Super foods

- Body Balance

- Osteoprocare

- Electrolife (www.AriseandShine.com)

- Super Ionic Minerals

- Organic Green Vegetables

Any other source made from either organic or wild greens that is not heated in any way, has no fillers or other toxins. This means you can't buy most things at a regular grocery store as they're not made from food usually, and if they are they tend to be heated "pasteurized" or have lots of fillers in them.

How much should you have? As much as you can! The only thing to watch for is if you go too fast you can experience diarrhea, a common cleansing reaction because minerals remove toxins. **So be sure to go slow at first and then keep increasing and increasing without limits** because the more you take the better.

Enjoy these minerals, your energy levels will skyrocket!

Chapter Five Inspired Actions

Choose any one or more of the following *Inspired Actions:*

- Read The 11 Must Haves: The Essential Nutrients Your Body Needs

- Order at least one of the mineral products above from (www.THMastery.com) or purchase them at your health food store.

- Read *The pH Miracle* By Dr. Robert Young Ph.D.

- Eat at least 1 organic green vegetable every day for one week

- Make Mineral Broth

- Order a juicer from www.THMastery.com and make tasty vegetable juices

Chapter Six
What To Eat

I said that I would tell you what I ate to cure myself of all of those "incurable" diseases. Well, now's the time. By the way, **I don't believe there is any such thing as an incurable disease.** You can choose to believe anything you want. I can only come from my experience. Since I can only come from my experience, I would ask you not to believe anything I say but rather keep an open mind and try out the things that you read here. If what I say works in the real world keep it and if it doesn't then get rid of it. I am more committed to your success than whether you believe anything I say or not. Again, I personally don't believe there is any such thing as an incurable disease.

What I ate when I first found perfect health for myself was about 95% fresh, organic fruits, vegetables, seeds and nuts along with some fresh organic green juice made in a Green Star juicer and about a table spoon of Vitamineral Greens every day. THAT'S IT!!! **I also told myself every day that I'm healthy, which is very important because the #1 factor in being healthy constantly are the thoughts you send throughout your body.** Even more surprising to you would be to know that if I knew then what I'm sharing with you in this book now, it would have been far easier (no cleansing reactions) and far faster, probably only a few weeks, not six months.

Naturally my intellect didn't believe it would work. My mind kept saying "but we have to eat meat for protein, everybody knows that" and "we need milk for calcium, everyone knows that." Fortunately for me my heart and my body were speaking louder than my mind long enough for me to read all of the books that showed me the science. Everything I've read scientifically has validated what actually works in the real world...which is why HUNDREDS OF THOUSANDS OF PEOPLE HAVE CURED THEMSELVES OF MANY ILLNESSES AND LOST WEIGHT just by eating fresh living organic foods.

"If this was true then everyone would know it!"

You may be thinking that now. But for a long time everyone knew the world was flat and that the Earth is the center of the universe and the sun goes around the Earth. We "knew it" that all knowledge was kept in the Canon (the Bible and the writings of Aristotle and Plato), that disease was caused by demons and we used leeches to suck out demons, that black people were less than white people, that women should not be allowed to vote, that we couldn't fly to the moon, that the car would never be affordable to the average person, that there is no such thing as electricity and so on and so on.

We as a civilization have believed a lot of totally ridiculous things. It often took great upheavals like our civil rights movement in America during the 1960's to awaken people to the truth. Fairly soon we will see the ideas that we need meats and dairy products for good health to be as the six time iron man winner and record holder Dave Scott says, "the ridiculous fallacies" that they are. We already know why we are so ingrained with false beliefs, the National Dairy Council provides all of our health education, and they have since 1915. They still visit our public schools today and continue to influence the minds of our young Americans. Did you learn in school that four time Mr. Universe, Bill Pearl, is like Dave Scott, Edwin Moses, Carl Lewis and so many more are vegetarians?

Here is a scientific fact that may shock you. As little as 50 milligrams of cooked food causes a toxic shock reaction in the body. Look it up in *Spiritual Nutrition* a book by Yale graduate Dr. Gabriel Cousens MD. The best foods for our body are fresh organic fruits and vegetables, seeds and nuts. These foods are higher in water, fiber, enzymes, minerals, vitamins, good fats, usable proteins and more. I cover every single nutrient in our trainings and in my book *The 11 Must Haves: The Essential Nutrients Your Body Needs.* I also give you many recipes, a full menu and teach you how to make up your own recipes. For now, I'm going to give you a few really potent weight loss recipes to get you started. Of course you can have as many salads, fruits and other living foods that you want. For more info on diet **see our FREE sample menu plan at** www.THMastery.com or pick up a copy of *The SuperStyle Diet Recipe Class Video or Book* where we not only have more recipes but more information on daily menu plans, supplements to take, tools you need for your kitchen and more.

Arnoux's Famous Chocolate Milkshake

For All You Chocolate Lovers!

- The Meat of 3 Young Coconuts
- The Milk of 1-3 Young Coconuts (add only enough to blend and then add more after blending until you have your choice of shake or milk)
- 1 T of Cacao Powder
- 1 *cap* full of Vanilla Extract or 1/2 of a vanilla bean
- 1-3 T of Raw Agave Nectar
- A dash of Celtic or Himalayan Sea Salt (regular sea salt or table salt is toxic (see *The Salt Conspiracy* by Victoria Bidwell) and ruins the taste)
- A heaping T of Vanilla flavored Nutritional Essentials (By Natural Choice Products)
- 1 T of OsteoProCare

Blend all of the ingredients with the milk from the young coconut and then add six or so ice cubes and bend again. Taste. If it's not better than your favorite chocolate drink you probably need more Agave sweetener. Share with everyone you know and send

43

them to www.THMastery.com for the FREE recipe! Enjoy!

Please note, add the liquid supplements after blending directly into the drink and stir. Most of the ingredients for all of these recipes can be found on our website as well. These recipes can be made without the supplements for those on a tighter budget, but they won't taste as well or be as powerful for weight loss.

The Weight Lifter's Dream

Fat Burner Supreme

- Milk and Meat of 3 Young Coconuts
- A dash of Celtic or Himalayan Sea Salt
- 1 - 2T Raw Agave Nectar or Honey
- 1t of a Super Green Powder (Such as Vitamineral Green or Tonic Alchemy)
- 1/2 of a Vanilla Bean or 1 cap full of Vanilla Extract A heaping T of Vanilla flavored Nutritional Essentials (By Natural Choice Products at www.THMastery.com.)
- 1 T of OsteoProCare (www.THMastery.com)

Blend all. The consistency will be creamy if you use a Vitamix or Total Blender. If you don't, these recipes may not taste as good so be sure to get a good blender ASAP. You may have small coconut chunks if you use a normal blender. We carry both blenders at www.THMastery.com.

Blend with ice cubes for extra chill. Try using coconut water iced cubes. It won't taste as good without ice! Please note, add the liquid supplements after blending directly into the drink and stir if possible.

Thai Coconut Soup

- Milk of 1 Young Coconut
- ½ t Celtic or Himalayan Sea Salt
- Dash of Agave Nectar or Honey
- Juice of 2-3 Limes (no seeds!)
- Fresh Jalapeno Pepper (try ¼ and see how hot it is - I like ¾ of a pepper)
- 3 Cucumbers
- Fresh Basil (to taste)
- 2 Scallions
- Lemon Grass (to taste)

(Blend above ingredients, use rest as garnish)

- Bean Sprouts
- 1 Avocado Cubed
- Cilantro

The Basic Green Smoothie

Do you remember the testimonials from Carmen Sanchez and Nurse Stephanie?

This was their secret to massive weight loss. This meal alone can be your staple meal replacement. MANY people have lost a lot of weight simply by replacing 5-10 meals per week with a green smoothie.

- 20% any vegetable such as spinach, celery, kale, etc
- 80% any fruit such as apple, orange, banana, mango, etc
- Add water

Blend, how simple! As time goes on you'll want more vegetables and less fruits naturally as your taste buds change. You'll never get bored because you can use any organic fruits or vegetables that you want. You can also add any of the supplements that we recommend. When you learn the secret of preparing gourmet foods from *The SuperStyle Diet Video or Book* or during our live trainings you'll love it even more! If all that you take from this book is making a green smoothie every day we will have effectively changed your life forever!

Again, as a reminder, It must be noted that ALL of these recipes are not as good if made in a standard blender. They should be done in a Total Blender or Vitamix found at www.THMastery.com.

Learning how to eat more living foods, more fresh organic fruits, vegetables, seeds and nuts is a real undertaking. Naturally, I recommend my seminar for that purpose but for now do the best you can. If you can eat 50% or more living foods you're going to be doing well. If you can do 80% you'll probably lose eight pounds per month on average. 100%? I wouldn't do it without guidance. You may have a hard time or detoxify too fast and get discourage, but the results will be mind blowing.

The goal is NOT to eliminate things from your diet but to add more and more good things little by little until your lifestyle has shifted. Don't diet, just add good things like green smoothies and over time you'll see fantastic results. Remember, what you resist persists and what you focus on expands. If you focus on adding in good things you'll get more of that.

Addiction

Food addiction is not to be taken lightly. In my experience, which is quite extensive in regards to addiction, food addiction is the toughest of all.

I have created a program to *eliminate all cravings* and make it possible for you to choose a healthy lifestyle that keeps you looking hot and sexy called *How to Overcome Addictions Without Willpower*, which I include in our live trainings. I am going to give you many of the tools that are part of the program in this book, hopefully enough to get you to your goals. You already have a few of them.

In the most basic terms, addiction is generally old programming, self-medicating or stuffing old feelings and physical toxins coming into the blood stream. The secret is to reprogram yourself, make yourself feel good and cleanse the toxins out before they hit your blood stream while giving yourself the proper nutrition. Making yourself feel good and reprogramming are so important to sticking with a diet or healthy lifestyle.

Let's begin to discover some secrets about that in the next chapter.

Chapter Six Inspired Actions

Choose any one or more of the following *Inspired Actions:*

- Make Arnoux's Famous Chocolate Milkshake

- Make a Green Smoothie

- Invest in a high quality blender (www.THMastery.com)

- Get *The SuperStyle Diet Recipe Class Video or Book* (www.THMastery.com)

- Choose a percentage of fresh, living or raw foods that you will eat each day and stick with it.

Chapter Seven
The Emotional Body

Many of us have been taught to keep our emotions in. That big boys or girls don't cry. That showing emotions shows weakness and so on. It's time to let those old ideas go as they don't work, they don't support us and they don't make us stronger. As a black belt and instructor under one of the world's greatest martial arts masters I learned that **a true warrior releases their emotions responsibly. We don't dump them on other people and we don't stuff them down inside.** We release them using very powerful and effective methods that allow us to finally be free of the weight we've been carrying: this is emotional weight, but it's also physical weight.

Emotions are chemicals. Every time you think a thought biochemicals are created in your brain that enter your body and allow you to feel the feelings you've created with your thoughts. This is a scientific fact that I learned in biology as a pre-med student at the University of Washington. It's well illustrated in a movie called *What the Bleep Do We Know?* These chemicals are highly toxic if they are unhappy emotions and if not released they stay in our cells causing illness *and* cause us to carry weight. Emotions may be the most important toxins to release, even more than undigested foods and environmental toxins. If you don't get the emotional toxins out of your fat cells they may never break down.

Many of us, especially women have sexual trauma in our history. This can be a big block to losing weight because becoming attractive can be scary on a subconscious level. **Releasing the emotions stuck in the body from the trauma can cause dramatic weight loss.**

There are many ways to release emotions like journaling, punching pillows, crying and so on. Most of these will NOT permanently release the emotion but will clear it out for the present moment. I created a method out of necessity that has changed my life and the lives of many others. Using this method that I call *The 7-Steps to Reprogramming Yourself,* I've been able to release emotions as they came up and that particular feeling never, ever comes back. When the emotion was causing a craving for food the craving went away!

I helped a participant in my seminar totally and permanently clear the anxiety she felt whenever she got down to a certain weight in twenty minutes. Another participant, Rachel Kane, on her own permanently cleared her fear of flying which was so severe she couldn't sleep the night before a scheduled trip! The stories of what people have done with this process are almost unbelievable. I've seen people clear anger, sadness, fear and any other emotion that exists. I've seen people release traumas of divorce or a bad break up, rape, molestation, verbal abuse, physical abuse, horrible childhood trauma, witnessing a death, the suicide of a loved one, and fears like fear of flying, heights, public speaking, singing, investing and even the fear of bugs! Sometimes even I get surprised, and I've seen a lot.

Check these stories out:

"I grew up with a less than perfect home life to say the least. A lot of my memories from my earliest days were full of fear and panic. I don't remember ever feeling safe. I tried many things to escape, but they didn't work. I finally realized something was wrong with me but I did not know how to fix it, so I spent thousands of dollars over a ten year period attending seminars, having sessions with various types of healers, reading books, and listening to tapes. I was determined to "be and feel normal." Nothing seemed to work.

Finally, I discovered Arnoux's class Total Health Mastery and learned *The 7-Steps to Reprogramming Yourself*. Within a few weeks of eating a fresh raw food diet and using his reprogramming technique almost every day, I felt a moment of peace. I remember contacting Arnoux at that moment, because I was so excited not to feel the underlying fear for what seemed to be the first time ever! Later, I had days of more peace and happiness and less fear and anxiety. I was calm and I wasn't doing anything else differently. It was amazing!!

Now a year later, I am comfortable with me... with my weight, with my personality, with me in general. I graduated from law school 10 years ago but went into sales rather than practice law, because I could not focus on one thing for very long. At the time I thought I just liked sales more than the practice of law, but looking back now, I think my short attention span was one of the effects of feeling so much fear so often.

After working with Arnoux, I am able to focus and feel good. I just passed the bar exam and am now practicing law and loving it!! I could go on and on about the magnificent changes that have occurred in my life since working with Arnoux... I had been single for many years and now I am dating. I am also enjoying my relationship with my friends and family so much more. Thank you Arnoux so much!!!"

- Mari Davis, Savannah, GA

"I was working with Arnoux on my weight and we were doing great losing ten pounds per month for several months. Then I was stuck. Nothing moved for three weeks. Several days later I shared with Arnoux a huge fear that had come up with me where I felt like a 15 years old. He asked what happened when I was 15 and I told him it was when I was raped but I had dealt with it in therapy already. He suggested that there was still something there and that he could help me clear it. In only a few minutes time we cleared some core beliefs that were associated with that trauma and I went to sleep. Believe it or not...I woke up five pounds lighter!!! Arnoux said the body holds emotions in the fat cells. Amazing. Thank you Arnoux!!!"

- Samara Christy, Health Care Practitioner, Scottsdale, AZ

"My whole life my mom has mentally and emotionally abused me. As an adult I had still been dealing with how angry and sad I was that I felt my mom didn't love me and hated me so much. All of the mean things she used to say to me kept repeating in my head. I was very depressed, drank a lot of alcohol, considered ending it many times or going on heavy meds. Arnoux taught me his *7-Steps to Reprogramming Yourself* but I didn't use it because it seemed too easy to work on something that intense and painful. Two years later he taught it to me again and I was really at the end of my rope so I tried it. Within a few weeks of using the 7-Steps I had cleared a lot of my sadness. Everyone at work, all of my friends and my sister were asking me what I did. So I'm teaching them this very simple process that ACTUALLY WORKS! I still have my anger to deal with, but now I know how to. Thanks Arnoux, you saved my life! Seriously, I don't know what I would've done without you."

- Nikki P., Nurse Practitioner, Seattle, WA

This process isn't just about releasing old emotions and subconscious thoughts that don't support you forever, it's also about ending repeating patterns in your life. Patterns of food addiction, of not exercising, of low self-esteem, of depression and any other type of negative pattern including those not related to health or weight loss. My friends, this technology has totally changed my life and allowed me to live my dreams! It can for you too so please, please, please master it and begin to do the same thing that so many others have done with it, FEEL BETTER!

Be aware, the #1 reason why people don't use it is the idea that they can't or that it won't work or that it's too good to be true. In our seminar we have you clear those blocks to using this technology during the course. I encourage you, no I strongly stand up and tell you with all of my heart and soul, PLEASE clear out any of those thoughts or feelings that it won't work for you right away! As soon as you finish this chapter!

One thing I love about this process is that you can do it yourself. You don't have to keep paying someone to guide you through the process. I also love the fact that you don't have to release the emotions consciously; they leave you on EVERY LEVEL including physical when you're sleeping. You may have dreams called "venting dreams" where you feel the emotions release during the dream. You may also have dreams about the new programs that you put into your subconscious. Not only do you release the old feelings forever, you also reprogram your subconscious mind, eliminate repeating thought patterns and that changes your life.

We go into great detail on how to use this process in our live trainings but you can do it on your own just from following the steps. Here they are:

The 7-Steps to Reprogramming Yourself

- **Step 1:** Get present to the feeling
- **Step 2:** Ask, "if this feeling could talk, what would it say?"
  (write down exactly what it says)
- **Step 3:** In cursive, write the EXACT opposite of what it says

Example

The feeling says: "*I'll never be thin.*"

You write in cursive: "*I'll never **not** be thin.*"

The exact opposite isn't necessarily a truthful statement. The exact opposite doesn't need to make grammatical sense. Simply add in the word "not" or "don't" or remove the words "not" while keeping the rest of the statement exactly as originally written.

- **Step 4:** Repeat steps two and three until the feeling is completely gone
- **Step 5:** Go back and for each "cancellation" write your new belief in cursive

Rules For Writing New Beliefs

- Be sure its written as a positive statement.
- Be sure it's written in the present tense.
- It must make you feel good.

EXAMPLE

The cancellation is: "*I'll never not be thin.*"
You write in cursive: "I have the body of my dreams."

- **Step 6:** Within thirty minutes of falling asleep at night read all of the cancellations and new beliefs. You can simply ignore what the feeling said (step #2) and just read the cancellation.

- **Step 7:** Check the next day to be sure that it is gone. If not, which happens about 1 in 1,000 times, there are two possible reasons. Most commonly you thought you got everything the feeling had to say and that it was gone, but it wasn't, you perhaps were just numb at that point. So the next day the rest of it became present. You'll know because there will be some new statements that it says. The other less common possibility is that your body couldn't process all of the emotion out in one night. Then you'll just read what you had again.

This is the most basic version of *The 7-Steps to Reprogramming Yourself.* There are 3 more advanced levels that are even faster. If it takes 1 hour to clear an emotion with this method here it would only take 40 minutes with the next advanced level and only 4 minutes with the third level and *only two minutes with the most advanced level*! We show you the next two advanced levels of how to do the 7-Steps in the book on *The 7-Steps to Reprogramming Yourself.* The most advanced method requires more training and is part of our Master level certification program for the 7-Steps.

If you are experiencing any problems having this incredible process work for you please consider taking our live trainings that include teaching this process. This process alone will certainly change your life. Using *The 7-Steps to Reprogramming Yourself* as emotions come up will eliminate the cravings that go with them and will allow you to move towards the body and level of health you deserve and this is of the utmost importance.

Chapter Seven Inspired Actions

Choose any one or more of the following *Inspired Actions:*

- Write a list of emotions that you feel don't support you that you have come up regularly, on occasion or that you feel right now.

- Try doing *The 7-Steps to Reprogramming Yourself* with one of your emotions, especially on any feelings about not being able to do it, or that it's too good to be true.

- Hire a Professional Health Consultant to help guide and support you with clearing old emotions using *The 7-Steps to Reprogramming Yourself* (www.THMastery.com)

- Read *The 7-Steps to Reprogramming Yourself* book (www.THMastery.com)

Chapter Eight
The Mental Body

Even after I was able to clear emotions as they came up I was still addicted to food. I didn't feel like I was, but I found myself *automatically* doing things that were not what I was committed to. The source of this behavior is subconscious programming.

This programming is old beliefs that are programmed in the subconscious mind. Beliefs like, "once you hit 40 it's all down hill from there." Or "there is no cure for cancer." Or some painful ones like, "I'm fat, ugly and stupid." You may not *consciously* believe any of it, but if it's programmed in, you'll act upon these old beliefs as if you were a machine, it's just automatic. You need to release or change them all. If you're not already aware of the negative thoughts you have, you can find them with *The 7-Steps to Reprogramming Yourself.* Another way you discover them is by noticing how it makes you feel when you do things that are not on the path to your dreams coming true. If you suddenly reach for a big bag of potato chips and down the whole bag in five minutes. How did that make you feel emotionally? It's connected to the old programs. Follow the feelings to the programming using The 7-Steps outlined in Chapter 7 and clear it out.

That is huge! **This is a very big secret of weight loss.** I had someone take my seminar because she wanted to lose weight. At one point I asked for a volunteer to clear something so everyone could see how it works. She volunteered. She was feeling a deep sadness. We cleared that. Underneath it was anger. Then more sadness and then finally a big fear; we cleared all of these layers. One huge belief associated with the fear, the last layer of emotion was: "If I don't clean my plate I'll get sick and my mom will get in trouble." A trauma from age four. She said she always cleaned her plate totally even if she was completely full or on a diet and couldn't make herself stop. She never understood why until that day. Everyone in the audience could see that having a program like that running subconsciously would make it hard for anyone to lose weight. Now it's your chance to discover your old programs and delete them forever. You now have the power! YES!

To change our behavior we can consciously force ourselves to do what is best for us or we can use our power and change the subconscious programs that cause us to repeat old patterns. It is much easier and more powerful to simply re-program ourselves to do the things that we want to do. We can even create our own new programs by writing a script and put it into our subconscious, greatly impacting our tendencies and desires to follow old habits if not totally wiping them out leaving us to choose consciously. I'll show you how to do this in a moment.

To effectively change our long standing habits which are programmed into our subconscious we must access the subconscious directly, bypassing the filter called "the Critical Mind" as explained by John Kappas author of "*Success is Not an Accident*". We must bypass this filter and put into our computer the programs we want to be our behavior. **We have access to our subconscious mind 30 minutes or less before we go to sleep.** Simply by writing in cursive or longhand before bed we can literally program into our minds anything we wish. Writing in print re-activates the critical mind, so be sure to write in cursive. This is also why the sixth step of The 7-Steps is to read the cancellations and new beliefs within 30 minutes of falling asleep at night.

This information can be used very powerfully to heal deep issues and repeating patterns in life and applies to money, sex, love, health and every other area of our life. Start today!

The 7-Steps is for pulling out negative programs or thoughts that keep repeating over and over subconsciously and replacing them with new positive programs or new beliefs. Amazingly it pulls out the negative emotions that are locked together with the beliefs that are in your body as well. It actually releases those emotions from your cells while you are asleep. There are other techniques designed simply to put positive programming into your subconscious mind. This technique puts in the positive new beliefs and more importantly removes the negative beliefs and feelings that were in the way of your success. In other books I'll discuss in greater details methods for creating what you want in life such as visualization and so on. Let me share one of the most powerful ones with you now.

Have you read the book *Think and Grow Rich* by Napoleon Hill? If not, please do read it right away. Napoleon was asked by one of the world's richest men, Dale Carnege to dedicate his life to discovering the patterns of self-made millionaires. The patterns of success. Napoleon took him up on his charge and he spent literally decades studying the wealthiest and most successful people in the world. He went and lived with great men like Thomas Edison who didn't just make a working light bulb but invented the beginnings of almost every technology we use today such as 35mm film, the movie camera, the movie studio, the light rail train, the electric car, a working phone (he took Alexander Graham Bell's invention and made it useful), the microphone, and the first device ever created that could record and play back sound, the phonograph. He actually made movies before the year 1900!

Napoleon also studied and stayed with Henry Ford, who made the car affordable to the average man and was one of the richest men in the world. He also studied other great financial successes like Dale Carnegie and finally he wrote his book.

In the book he says that there is only one secret of being rich. That all rich people use it and those that don't, don't get rich. He mentions many other great strategies and tools, but continues to emphasize this one secret. What is the secret? Write down your intention or goal that you want to create as if it is already real (positive present tense) and read it every night before bed and every morning until every cell in your body believes it is true.

Well, if it works for getting rich why not use it for weight loss? I'm going to show you how! Keep in mind that you must write it in cursive for it to access your subconscious mind and that you must keep reading it every night until it comes true. Dr. John Kappas taught us that every time we put a positive program in it pushes out a little bit of the many negative programs that contradict it. If we keep putting a positive program in eventually it will push out all of the negative blocks and the goal will come true.

To begin changing your weight and health programs write your own paragraph or longer "script" in cursive that you will **read to yourself every night before bed** and every morning when you wake up. It'll just take a *minute* each day. Your script can be the generic one below, but writing your own in your words from your heart is very powerful. All you need to do is say what you don't like or don't want anymore and what you do like now and what you do want. This is how we create new programs and put them in. It doesn't directly remove old programs like The 7-Steps does, but if you keep putting the new program in, the same one, it eventually pushes out any conflicting old programs. Once this happens and your subconscious, conscious and the cells of your body are 100% totally aligned with your new program, then, and ONLY then will it become reality for you! So keep reading it morning and night until it is your reality. You can speed up the process anytime by using The 7-Steps to remove any negative programs that you find.

For example, "I love eating a diet of 70% organic fresh fruits and vegetables.. I love to exercise every day. I wake up early just before my alarm full of energy and vitality. I feel better and better every day. I am at my perfect weight. I feel amazing!"

How did that make you feel reading that? Wouldn't you like to write your own? Well now is the time, get to it. Grab a pen and paper! You may include other areas of health as well such as sleeping, breathing, relaxing, shopping, food preparation, etc.

After you've got it the way you want you can write it in cursive beautifully on a 3x5 card or nice piece of paper to read each night and morning until you achieve your goals and the intentions you are reading have become part of your life. Reading it in the mirror is very, very powerful and highly recommended. Be sure to visualize with all five senses what you are reading and creating. While you're imagining your goal be sure to see, hear, taste, feel and smell everything you are creating. Pay attention to how you feel the next day and as the days go by and you'll see the power of what you are doing here.

One thing you may be wondering is, "what if I don't feel good about my goals? What if every time I read them I feel depressed, upset, angry or afraid? Then what?" Take a deep breath and know that you have a great opportunity in front of you. You've just found some of the stuff blocking you from achieving those goals. Simply use The 7-Steps and release all of the negative emotions and beliefs coming up until you do feel good about your goals. This will skyrocket you to realizing them!

Your New You Picture

Reprogramming beliefs isn't all of it. There is also your self-image.

We all have an image in our mind of what we look like. **Our subconscious mind will automatically cause us to do the things we need to do so that we can look like that image.** What we do to change it is actually quite easy. Take a picture of your face and tape it onto your ideal body and put it somewhere that you can see it before falling asleep at night.

The best selling book of all time (besides the Bible) is called *Chicken Soup for the Soul* by Mark Victor Hansen and Jack Canfield. In the book they mention this exact same thing. They go on to say that using this one simple exercise caused one of them to lose 35lbs in less than two months!

If you see yourself as thin, healthy, sexy, buff, whatever you want on the inside, it will eventually become so on the outside. This is a great secret of life. T. Harv Eker, author of the #1 NY Times best seller *Secrets of the Millionaire Mind* says, "If you want to change the fruits go to the roots." The inner world creates the outer world. If you'd like to go to one of Harv's introductory evenings, *The Secret Psychology of the Millionaire Mind*, please visit our website www.THMastery.com.

The Conscious Mind

You must believe in yourself. You must believe consciously that you can lose weight. That you *can* do it. That you deserve to look beautiful, handsome, sexy and be healthy, all of it. Be very careful, watch your thoughts and make sure that you really believe in yourself and what is possible. Do NOT listen to anyone who tells you that you can't. **There is no such thing as can't** when we are talking about your potential. You CAN do anything. When Henry Ford said that he was going to make the automobile affordable to the average person everyone laughed at him. One of his famous quotes is, "if you think you can or you think you can't, either way you're right." He was great friends with Thomas Edison who was told many times that he can't. That he can't create a light bulb that will last. But he did. You too will do what others think isn't possible, *if you believe* you can. No doctor that I went to thought I could ever heal. They were wrong. Do not argue with those who don't believe in you, simply wish them well and keep going. What you resist persists. Unconditional love and acceptance is the only way to transcend naysayers. The proof is in the pudding so don't try to convince anyone with words. **Just do it and then they'll be begging you to show them how. You'll be a leader that way**.

Here are a few more tips and tools to help you succeed. What would happen if you did them all? What would that say about the kind of person you are? Good things for sure!

Your Environment

Your environment plays a big role in your success on a healthy weight loss program. Beware of the naysayers as even those that have good intentions may not have the knowledge that you now do. You don't have to tell people what you are up to! Choose people who believe in your unlimited potential. Watch out for commercials. Hit mute!

Collage

Put up a collage of your goal. Create beautiful images drawn or cut out, words and pictures that describe the goal already accomplished. This is a VERY powerful exercise. If you aren't sure that you want to do this watch a movie called *The Secret*. It will help you to realize your potential and your dreams.

Support Group or Buddy

To help you on your journey I recommend a support group or a buddy. Get around people at least once a week that encourage and inspire you to stick with your program. There are many, find one that works for you. Or you can find someone to be your buddy. To have a healthy dinner with you once a week or have a check-in call every day. This will make a world of difference.

Finally, the biggest secret of controlling your environment and inspiring you to success.

When I healed myself from all of those nasty illnesses I was living in a home where delicious smelling cooked foods were being made every day. For most people the temptation of homemade food would have been too much and they wouldn't have been able to stick with the program. That would have been true for me too except for this one secret. *At every meal I read about living foods.* Every single one without fail. Breakfast, lunch and dinner. I would have a craving for ice cream and start reading about how eating living foods cuts on average two hours off of our sleep time, gives us great energy and will heal my body and then I would notice I really liked watermelon a lot more than ice cream! This was my saving grace and now it can be yours. Read about health!

A few books I recommend:

- *Cleanse and Purify Thyself* by Dr. Richard Anderson
- *Diet for a New America* by John Robbins
- *The Miracle of Fasting* by Dr. Paul Bragg, PhD

Even if all you do is read for five minutes per day it will make a difference. Another alternative is to get the *Total Health Mastery 10-Week Seminar* audio or other audios and videos that support you.

Written words by a credible source have far more weight or impact than commercials, billboards, naysayers and anything else in the environment around you. Try it out. Reprogram your subconscious mind including your self-image, create a positive environment to support you and you will be well on your way.

Chapter Eight Inspired Actions

Choose any one or more of the following *Inspired Actions:*

- Read *Think and Grow Rich* by Napoleon Hill

- Read *Success is Not an Accident* By Dr. John Kappas

- Read any other book I recommended on health

- Create a "new you" picture with your face on your ideal body and place it somewhere that you'll see it every night before bed.

- Write down your weight loss goals in cursive and read them every night and every morning until you achieve them. If they upset you use *The 7-Steps to Reprogramming Yourself* to clear the upset and feel better.

- Create a Collage

- Find a weight loss buddy

- Every morning look in the mirror and say three nice things to yourself and keep going until you feel good. If you start crying you need to do this. Use The 7-Steps to clear away any pain that may come up.

Chapter Nine
The Spiritual Body

In science we learn that everything is made of atoms, constantly moving atoms. Everything, even solid objects are moving on the inside. **Everything is made of energy,** some moving faster than others. Einstein's E=MC squared only says that energy equals mass moving at the speed of light multiplied by itself. In plain English, if mass moves fast enough it becomes energy, if energy moves slow enough it becomes mass. Even fat cells. That's why we talk about this, because old heavy energy also becomes physical weight.

There are simple and easy ways to clear energy that I will share with you. There are more advanced ways of clearing energy meant for other books. The basics of clearing away old energy are based in the four elements, Earth, Air, Water and Fire, as well as Sound and Prayer.

Water

Water is a powerful purifier. It simply washes away old energy. Don't you feel refreshed after a hot shower? I do. Nothing can replace a dip in the ocean. I recommend you take a nice bath in purified water for an hour every day for one week to feel just how powerful it is. You will definitely feel relaxed. Taking two showers a day is a good idea as well. You can order a shower filter from us if you don't have one already. It's a very important investment in your health as the human body absorbs 100 times more cancer causing chlorine through the skin than if we drink it.

Fire

Have you ever felt joyful after sitting around a campfire? Fire burns away old energy. Wood fires, non-toxic candles and sunshine all are sources of fire. When you're taking your hot bath light some candles for fire.

Air

Breathing is a beautiful gift. Breathing is the most important involuntary function of the body that we can easily and actively control. Every conscious breath releases old energy. In Latin the word spirit and the word breath are the same word. When you breathe go in and out through the nose and breathe down below your belly button. Don't force, but rather relax and allow the breath to softly find its way down to your power center, below your belly button. Try taking 10 deep breaths outdoors three times per day to get centered and let go of old energy.

Earth

Earth is connecting with the beauty of Mother Nature. Appreciating the beauty of flowers, trees, mountains and so on allows us to connect, and let go of the old. Earth also includes touch. Touch is vital to life. Babies that are not held can die from lack of touch. This is still true when you're an adult, you need physical touch. If you don't have a lover get a massage at least once a week. If you can't afford it then consider bartering or a trade. Also, enjoy walking on grass, dirt or sand barefoot.

Sound

Singing is a great release. Continue to sing in the shower or in your car, or get your own Karaoke machine!

Deep Relaxation

Deep relaxation is giving the mind a break by focusing on a single thing such as your breath. A simple relaxation technique is to just keep on paying attention to your breathing, if thoughts pop up, keep breathing. Try fifteen minutes per day to start, and if you find it's really making a difference go to an hour. This practice is scientifically proven in to make you smarter, younger, calmer and happier. Try it out.

Prayer

If you believe in the power of prayer, which is highly documented, then please pray that you will be thin. If you don't believe in prayer, then simply visualize yourself thin every single morning and night while you read your goals for at least five minutes. It's easy and when you begin to truly see, feel and believe yourself to be the ideal weight that you want to have, then you will finally begin to have it.

Commitment

If you are not committed to yourself, your health, your dreams and your weight loss goals then they won't be achieved. You must be committed and dedicated. Do whatever it takes. Be unstoppable. Go for it! Apply everything in this book. Read it twice. Do ALL of the inspired actions and more. Go all the way and don't hold back and you will achieve your goals. I believe in you.

Chapter Nine Inspired Actions

Choose any one or more of the following *Inspired Actions:*

- Register for *The Solution Weekend Training* and put the dates in your day planner. Buy your plane tickets and book your hotel stay if you need to. See page 91 for details. Purchase the CD's or DVD's if you cannot attend live.

- Purchase *The Total Health Mastery 10-Week Seminar* as an audio, video or webinar right now without hesitation. Be totally committed to yourself, get the absolute best health education program available in the world today. (www.THMastery.com)

- Sit for 15 minutes every day and simply breathe

- Visualize yourself daily as having the body of your dreams, really let yourself feel that it is real

- Pray for your success with your health and weight

- Read *The 11 Must Haves: The Essential Nutrients Your Body Needs* to learn more about air, water, sunshine, and more

- Hire a Professional Health Consultant to help guide you and support you in achieving your weight loss goals (www.THMastery.com)

- Read this book again until you understand everything and have applied it. Consider taking on all of the inspired actions as they are designed to support you.

- Create a gratitude journal. Every night write at least five things that you are grateful for and allow yourself to truly feel the emotion. This alone can change your life. Try it for one week.

The Secrets

In the long run, losing weight doesn't happen with a pill. Losing weight comes from balancing the entire self. When you are healthy physically, emotionally, mentally and spiritually you will also be the ideal body that you desire. I hope that I have imparted to you the knowledge that has helped countless people create perfect health and the body of their dreams.

Now that you know what to do it's up to you. You have the power now, go for it!

To your amazing health!
Arnoux Goran

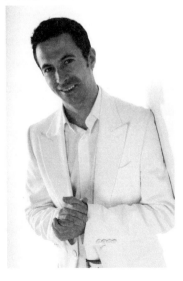

Arnoux (are-know) Goran has been studying health and healing for over 15 years and has earned 8 health related certifications. He is a renowned speaker and the author of the seven-book life changing series, *Total Health Mastery, The Total Health Mastery 10-Week Seminar, The Solution Weekend Seminar* and the Total Health Mastery Seminar Series. His passion for health grew after he cured himself of what were considered several incurable diseases and his doctors telling him "you won't be around much longer". He was diagnosed with arthritis, chronic fatigue syndrome, fibromyalgia, candida, ulcers, internal bleeding, severe allergies, asthma, hypoglycemia, anemia, total adrenal failure and more. He has lived in better than perfect health for nearly a decade now and has witnessed many people heal themselves from supposedly "incurable" diseases during The Total Health Mastery Seminars including cancer, diabetes, obesity, heart disease, high blood pressure, depression and more.

Acknowledgements

Firstly, I would like to thank God and all of the amazing support I have received in creating this book and all of our programs. When it was clear to me that my life was to be dedicated to teaching people about health and spirituality I had no idea that I would be so fulfilled and so inspired by the multitudes of people curing themselves of incurable diseases, losing weight when nothing else had worked, releasing addictions forever including food addictions, and that I would be the discoverer of one of the world's fastest and easiest method to permanently release old emotions and re-program the subconscious mind. I am so eternally grateful, thank you God.

I would like to thank my parents, my family, and all of my friends for your amazing support, love and care. I wouldn't have survived without you, much less live a life that I love.

Thanks to all of the participants of our seminars, your incredible dedication to yourself, your willingness to be responsible for your own health and well being and then applying the knowledge has truly inspired me. Every one of you who has accomplished the impossible through our programs, curing yourself of whatever you were afflicted with, thank you so much for sharing your success with me. It's because of you that our programs are growing so quickly and you're the reason why we work so hard to reach more people.

To the employees of *Total Health Mastery*, contractors, volunteers and everyone who has been working so hard to build this organization, I thank you from the bottom of my heart. Our Mission is being fulfilled and our Vision for the world is becoming more real every day. Thank you for creating with me.

To all of the Professional Health Consultants and Seminar Leaders of Total Health Mastery, thank you so much for being my partners in "creating a world of health". You are all so incredible, brilliant and true healers. That's worth everything.

Thank you to Rita Robinson and the others who contributed to this book.

Thank you to Chris McClary for doing a fantastic job on our corporate branding and book covers.

Finally, to my biggest supporter through the process of writing this book and in my life over the past two years, my editor, sweet love and wife, Lynn. You have been there for me in so many countless ways with love, care and wisdom. I've never been so supported and loved by anyone in my life. You are the best woman and I love you so much! I am so grateful to God that you are in my life and I cannot appreciate you enough for your loving support in every area of our lives.

Your FREE Bonus Included With This Book: *The Awakening*

Are you angry? Tired? In pain? Would you like to have more energy? Or be thinner? When I was young I had severe allergies. At age 13 I was in the ER because I couldn't breathe. At 16 my doctor said I had arthritis. By the age of 22 I was depressed and exhausted. I couldn't function without 12 hours of sleep. I had been diagnosed with ulcers, intestinal bleeding, asthma, total adrenal failure and worse. I was told if you don't do something different soon, you won't be around much longer. After trying every type of doctor I finally discovered what to do. By following the information from some new scientific health breakthroughs by the next spring I did not have a single thing wrong with me. No pain. No bleeding. No runny nose. My energy was high. My memory was back. I was healed! Since then I've made it my sole mission in life to share with others how I recovered and to help the world achieve what I so desperately needed, perfect health. The result is *The Awakening*.

To redeem your FREE audio version ($97 value) of this training please go to www.THMastery.com and keyword search *The Awakening*.

Total Health Mastery Presents:
The Solution Weekend Training

Would you like to have more energy?

What would your life be like if you needed two hours less sleep per night?

Would you like to lose weight, be more beautiful or simply feel better?

Are you afraid that someday you'll get Cancer? That you'll die of a horrible illness and suffer along the way? Are you dealing with fatigue, pain, obesity, depression or other health challenges?

You're not alone! America is facing a massive health epidemic. In the year 1900 1 in 16 Americans died of cancer, in 1970 it was 1 in 5 and now it is 1 in 4 people will die of a horrible cancer death! Currently the only treatments legally allowed, Chemotherapy, Radiation and Surgery provide a 2-3% success rate, the same as if you do nothing. But it's more than cancer. USA Today reported that 75% of Americans are in chronic pain. Currently 70% of Americans are overweight and 30% are obese. Obesity in adolescents has tripled over the last 20 years. Nearly half of Americans will die of a heart attack or a stroke. The number of Americans on Anti-depressants has doubled in the past 10 years. The rates of babies born Autistic have also tripled over the last decade. Childhood diabetes is skyrocketing.

EVERY American will develop a degenerative disease by the age of 40!

During *The Solution* Weekend Training presented by *Total Health Mastery* we will examine the current health epidemic and not only the impact on our daily lives both physically and emotionally, but the massive economic cost. We currently spend 15% of our production on health care yet remain the most unhealthy country in the world!

We will explore WHY these epidemics have broken out. It will be one of the most shocking and freeing experiences of your life!

And finally, a new hope will emerge for you as we unveil the new medical discoveries that have been made allowing for you to create levels of health never thought possible before. Once you begin on the path of health, lose weight, increase your energy levels and produce other results as seen in our five minute video on our website, YOU will be THE SOLUTION.

Register now at www.THMastery.com

Available Mini-Seminars

In Person or Via-Teleconference

- *The Solution Weekend Training*
- *An Introduction to Total Health Mastery™* (the audience shares what they want to learn about)
- *How to Overcome Addictions Without Willpower™*
- *How to Stop Emotional Eating™*
- *How to Cleanse the Body Without Cleansing Reactions™*
- *Why You Don't Lose Weight and How You Can™*
- *How to Skyrocket Your Energy Levels in 15 Minutes or Less™*
- *So You Think You Have an Incurable Disease?™*
- *Secrets of the World's Top Athletes™*
- *The SuperStyle Diet Recipe Class™* (Requires Fee For Food – Limited Availability – In Person Only in California)

The Total Health Mastery
10-Week Seminar

Have you ever been sick, overweight, tired or angry?

Millions of people around the world are suffering from disease, fatigue and emotional distress without solution or support.

The Total Health Mastery 10-Week Seminar provides a complete and advanced health education. Others who have taken our course via tele-conference, recording or in person have reported that they have:

- Overcome Addictions Without Willpower
- Removed Cellulite, Heavy Metals and other Toxins
- Stopped Emotional Eating
- Reversed Aging signs such as Wrinkles, Skin Blemishes and Hair Loss
- Discovered What You Need to Know about Diabetes, Cancer, Heart Disease, Autism and Arthritis
- Lost Weight Easily Even if Nothing Has Worked in the Past

- Learned the Secrets of the Worlds Greatest Athletes
- Released Old Emotions Permanently
- Learned to Reprogram the Subconscious Mind and Change Habits Forever
- Created a Healthy Body and Mind and Achieved Total Health Mastery

Attendees of our program consistently with our information and unique support system create unbelievable levels of health. The following represents just a FEW of our common testimonials:

"My wife Susan brought me here and at first I didn't want to have anything to do with it. I have a friend who is a vegetarian and five months ago I used to give him a bad time about it. I used eat steak and potatoes and I am from Montana. I have been on an 85-90% living food diet for the past 3 months and I have lost 30 plus pounds. I have pants that my wife told me to throw away a year ago that I am wearing now. When I started the course I was a size 44 and now I am a size 40. The main reason I got into this course was I had talked to Arnoux about my insulin. My pancreas was removed due to an accident. Now my insulin in-take is half of what it

used to be. My relationship with my wife is good. My energy is up, I sleep less and I'm going to take the class again because I know I missed so much the first time. Thank you Arnoux!" - Odin Myhre Huntington Beach, CA

"When I first started I was curious about health, and what our body does. Two major things happened: I used to take Xanex everyday to go to sleep because I had so much anxiety, and now I go to sleep right away. That was huge for me, and I never thought that would have had anything to do with my health. My broken heart... I had gone through a break up. I didn't know this class dealt with emotional stuff. I got over a broken heart that I had been trying to get over for a year. I've checked myself everyday now for the past month to see if it is really gone, because I just can't believe it. That alone is worth every bit of this course." - Jennifer Montanez Newport Beach, CA

"For as long as I can remember I have dealt with some kind of sickness in my life. It started when I was a baby and my Mom began then to look for

ways to heal me. This is the first time I have found anything that has made me feel better, everything else had made me feel "not as bad". Through this course I found hope that things can actually be great in my life and that I can feel really well. A few things that happened after just the first week; by just adding a green smoothie including oil, my skin became smooth and was no longer dry. Four or five weeks into it I noticed that my belt was one notch tighter. I am more graceful with myself and I am learning to let my feelings come. Feeling my feelings was a daunting task and now I have really learned how to do it."

Joy Hansen, Oakland, CA

Our 10-session seminar consists of 10 two-hour sessions. You may attend *anytime* via recording.

Some of the benefits of *The Total Health Mastery 10-Week Seminar* that others who have taken it have reported:

- Education about how to lose weight, how to eliminate cravings, how to reduce or eliminate pain or inflammation, how to create perfect skin, a more radiant glow and how to achieve perfect health forever.

- Learned how to permanently release old feelings from the past that wouldn't leave, how to change negative thinking overnight and finally achieve your goals.

- Greater self-confidence, motivation and zest for life! (Please note, we cannot promise anyone will achieve any of these results, but we can share what some of our former clients have shared with us.)

Our mission is to provide this education for EVERONE on planet Earth. **I believe when everyone on the planet knows the information contained in *The Total Health Mastery 10-Week Seminar*, sickness on the planet will end and never return.**

To find out more or to order visit www.THMastery.com

Host A Free Home Health Party!

Would you like to introduce the power of Total Health Mastery to your friends, family, office or church? Our professionally trained certified seminar leaders are ready and waiting to come to your home, office or any other meeting place to present a FREE mini-seminar, *The Awakening* for those that you love. **Not only will it change their lives forever, but you just may save a life!**

Even if they've tried everything they'll finally get the answers they're looking for. This is a great and amazing way to change the lives of the ones you love and make a HUGE impact on your community.

To host a home health party or corporate mini-seminar in your area simply call our office at 1-877-680-8200 and get scheduled. We will send you our promotional kit that includes everything you need to let everyone know about your party including our step-by-step guide to success as the host, flyers and an email to forward. You'll even get a script to guide you on what to say when you invite people.

These events are FREE (in California) and last two hours. We'll show them video testimonials of people who cured themselves of cancer, diabetes, obesity, depression and a lot more. No matter what they will be incredibly inspired and they will be forever touched and changed by your gift to them.

Call now us right now and schedule your first home health party or corporate mini-seminar. 1-877-680-8200.

totalhealthmastery

List Your Weight and Health Goals:

List old negative programs or emotions that you want to permanently clear using *The 7-Steps to Reprogramming Yourself*:

List each completed inspired action and the positive results:

Notes Section:

Notes Section: